Lose 90 Pounds in 3 Months:

Completely Change Your Body In Just 90 Days
Fitness Challenge

Table of content

Introduction

I would like to thank and congratulate you on downloading my book **"Lose 90 Pounds in 90 Days!"** Just by downloading this book you have shown me that you are ready to make some positive changes in your lifestyle. By improving your diet and introducing a healthy form of exercise into your life are going to combine to make your life light up in a positive way where you are going to feel and look younger and more vibrant than you have in a long time. This is the beginning of a new happier healthier way of living for you. You will have all the offered information within these pages to help give you support during your journey from healthy recipes, meal planner, exercises to try, and what you can do to help get the extra boost you need mentally on those hard days.

You want to stay in a positive mindset because that will make your transformation much easier, but reality is sometimes we all have those days when we need some extra support to get through them. You will have lots of supportive suggestions within these pages. I wish you a great read that will hopefully inspire you enough that you are ready and willing to take the 90 challenge to lose 90 pounds. Of course you may not be wanting to lose that much, you can adjust your daily diet to suit your specific needs—the foods included in this book are simply healthy foods that will only do you good—and benefit your health—so how can you go wrong?

Part 1. Recipes & 14 Day Meal Planner

List of the World's Healthiest Foods:

Vegetables:

- Asparagus
- Avocados
- Beets/Beet greens
- Bell peppers
- Bok Choy
- Broccoli
- Brussels sprouts
- Cabbage
- Carrots
- Collard Greens
- Corn
- Cucumbers
- Cauliflower
- Celery
- Potatoes
- Romaine Lettuce
- Sea vegetables
- Spinach
- Squash, summer
- Squash, winter
- Sweet potatoes
- Swiss Chard
- Tomatoes
- Turnip greens

- Eggplant
- Fennel
- Garlic
- Green Peas
- Green beans
- Kale
- Leeks
- Mushrooms crimini
- Mushroom Shiitake
- Mustard greens
- Olive oil, extra virgin
- Olives
- Onion

Seafood:

- Cod
- Tuna
- Shrimp
- Scallops
- Salmon
- Sardines

Eggs & Dairy:

- Eggs, pasture raised
- Cow's milk, grass fed
- Yogurt, grass-fed
- Cheese, grass-fed

Nuts & Seeds:

- Walnuts
- Sunflower seeds
- Sesame seeds
- Pumpkin seeds
- Peanuts
- Flaxseeds
- Cashews
- Almonds

Grains:

- Whole Wheat
- Rye
- Quinoa
- Oats
- Millet
- Buckwheat
- Brown rice
- Barley

Poultry & Meats:

- Beef, grass-fed
- Turkey, pasture raised
- Lamb, grass-fed
- Chicken, pasture raised

Beans & Legumes:

- Tofu
- Tempeh
- Soybeans
- Black beans
- Dried peas
- Garbanzo beans (chickpeas)
- Kidney beans
- Lentils
- Lima beans

- ♦ Miso
- ♦ Navy beans
- ♦ Pinto beans
- ♦ Soy Sauce

World's Healthiest Herbs & Spices:

- ◆ Chili pepper, dried
- ◆ Basil
- ◆ Black pepper
- ◆ Cinnamon
- ◆ Cloves
- ◆ Dill
- ◆ Ginger
- ◆ Cilantro & Coriander
- ◆ Oregano
- ◆ Mustard seeds
- ◆ Rosemary
- ◆ Peppermint
- ◆ Cumin Seeds
- ◆ Parsley
- ◆ Tumeric
- ◆ Thyme
- ◆ Sage

Fruits:

- ◆ Apricots
- ◆ Apples
- ◆ Watermelon
- ◆ Strawberries
- ◆ Raspberries
- ◆ Pears

- Prunes
- Cranberries
- Grapes
- Kiwl
- Oranges
- Figs
- Plums
- Lemon/limes
- Cantaloupe
- Bananas
- Blueberries
- Pineapple

Foods We Shouldn't Eat/Alternative Cheat Day Choices

◆ **Starbucks' Double Chocolaty Chip Frappuccino Blended Creme with Whipped Cream**—you will receive over half of a day's saturated fat from this drink as well as one-third of the maximum fat you should consume in a day. One 16-ounce drink is 510 calories, 19g fat, 11g saturated fat, 59g sugar, and 300 sodium.

Another Choice: Choose to go with a regular coffee without all the added extras. If you have a craving for a Frappuccino choose a light blended coffee that is around 130 calories, 0.5g fat, and 16g sugar.

◆ **Auntie Anne's Jumbo Pretzel Dog.** For the hotdog and pretzel lovers, this is a jumbo hotdog wrapped up in a pretzel bun—this food item is almost half of your daily upper limit of fat and sodium. One Jumbo pretzel dog with butter has wrapped up inside it 610 calories, 29g fat, 13g saturated fat, and 1,150 sodium.

Another Choice: Reduce your treat down to about 310 calories and only one gram of fat. Choose the original pretzel minus the butter.

◆ **Cinnabon's Caramel Pecanbon.** The smell of these yummy buns floating through the mall can be a real attraction for every sweet-tooth. These buns deliver about half the calories and just about all the fat you should consume in a day. One bun is 1,092 calories, 56g fat, and 47g sugar.

Another Choice: Why not choose to go with a Mini-bun, that are for smaller and smarter appetites, these are around 300 calories and 11g fat.

◆ **Wendy's Sweet and Spicy Boneless Wings.** There is a lot of salt in this dish, far too much for what you should be taking in for a day. When it comes to calories it is not bad in that area, as long as they are going to be your entire meal, minus any side dishes. One order of wings has 550 calories, 18g fat, 27g sugar, and a whopping 2,530 sodium.

Another Choice: Check out this tasty meal, a grilled chicken breast on a sesame-seed bun is 320 calories, seven grams of fat, eight grams of sugar, and 950 milligrams of sodium.

◆ **Dunkin Donuts' Coffee Cake Muffin.** You can choose to have this one muffin or you could have three glazed doughnuts instead—they will be equal in calories and nutrients. One muffin is 620 calories, 25g fat, 7g saturated fat, 54g sugar, and 93 carbs.

Another Choice: When you are looking for a sweet treat on a cheat day, you will be better off going with the glazed doughnut, as it has 220 calories, 9g fat, 12g sugar, and 31g carbs.

◆ **Olive Garden's Grilled Shrimp Caprese.** Shrimp a yummy tasting treat, and is low-fat, low-cal, high in protein and iron. But where you will start racking up the calories is with the garlic-butter sauce. The garlic-butter will use up your daily fat and about half of your sodium limit. One plate is 900 calories, 41g fat, and 3,490mg sodium.

Another Choice: Melted cheese and with marinara sauce on the side, is a lighter version to check out. Another option you might want to consider is the Venetian Apricot Chicken, it contains one-third the calories and 1/10 the fat, put still has a large amount of sodium.

◆ **Amy's Organic Thai Coconut Soup.** One serving of this soup is more than half of your daily limit of saturated fat and a quarter of your sodium. One half a can serving has 140 calories, 10g fat, 8g saturated fat, and 580mg of sodium.

Another Choice: Try Amy's lentil vegetable soup it is low-sodium, and is filled with veggies and protein, but with less fat and sodium: 4g fat, 0.5g saturated fat, and 340mg sodium.

◆ **Bear Naked Chocolaty Cherry Grain-ola Bar.** This bar is almost the same nutritional stats as Hershey's Sweet and Salty Reese's Peanut Butter bar. You could eat almost three Nature Valley Oats and Honey granola bars for the same intake. One 54-gram bar has 230 calories, 10g fat, and 14g sugar.

Another Choice: Barbara's Crunch Organic Oats and Honey Granola Bar with two bars only having 190 calories, 8grams of fat, and 10 grams of sugar.

◆ **Quaker Natural Granola, Low-Fat.** Some types of granola contain a large amount of sugar. This one has 18g of sugar. A 2/3 cup serving would have 210 calories, 3g fat, 4g protein, 3g fiber and 18g sugar.

Another Choice: Have a 2/3cup of Health Valley's Low-Fat Date Almond Flavor Granola with 180 calories, 1g fat, 10g sugar, 5g protein, and 6g fiber.

◆ **Vitamin Water.** Each bottle contains 2.5 servings of sugar-sweetened water, so a whole bottle delivers 33 g of sugar.

Another Choice: New vitamin water 10 only has 10 calories per serving or 25 per bottle and it contains zero-calorie sweeteners.

◆ **Healthy Choice Sweet and Sour Chicken.** The calories are not bad in this meal but the sugar and sodium are high, and it has more fat than most other Healthy Choice options. One meal has 400 calories, 13g protein, 5g fiber—but 10g fat, 20g sugar and 500mg of sodium.

Another Choice: The oven roasted chicken meal which has 260 calories, 5g fat, 9g sugar, 520mg sodium, 15g protein, and 6g of fiber.

◆ **PowerBar Performance Energy Cookies & Cream.** This power bar has only 1g of fiber and nearly three-fourths of the upper limit of daily added sugar. One bar is 240 calories, 26g sugar, 45g carbs, 8g protein, less than 1g of fiber.

Another Choice: Choose the PowerBar Harvest line of bars. These are made with whole grains, one oatmeal raisin cookie bar is 250 calories, 43g of carbs, 22g sugar, but has 10g protein and 5g fiber, vitamins, and minerals.

◆ **Kellogg's Pop-Tarts Brown Sugar Cinnamon.** If you eat both tarts this will give you a quarter of your daily fat, and more than half your added sugar for the day. Two pastries are 420 calories, 16g fat, 26g sugar and 66g carbs.

Another Choice: Eat only one pastry. You can also try Fiber One's Brown Sugar Cinnamon Toaster Pastry it has 190 calories, 4g fat, 16g sugar, 36g carbs and 5 fiber.

◆ **Coleslaw.** Coleslaw can lead you to believe it would be a good choice while dieting. But the average portion of coleslaw will have at least 260 calories, and more than 20g of fat, popular brands such as KFC's contains close to 26g of saturated fat making it worse than a portion of french fries.

Another Choice: Make it yourself using a fat free yogurt or reduced fat mayonnaise, create a healthier version that will taste great. You can spice up the flavor using lemon juice or vinegar.

◆ **Packaged Sandwiches.** Sandwiches that are already packaged usually contain large amounts of calories on average of 400 calories. They also contain large amounts of fat and saturated fat.

Another Choice: It is best to make your own sandwiches with a wholemeal bread, healthy salad, vegetables, and a light dressing. Add lean meat or you could choose to have a healthy veggie soup for lunch or egg on toast.

◆ **Tomato Sauce for Pasta or Chili.** Often these premade sauces are packed with refined sugars, promoting weight gain.

Another Choice: You can make a sauce that is simple to prepare and low on sugar and fat. Add a small amount of olive oil in pan, chop onion and add. Add a teaspoon of garlic, minced, one can of chopped tomatoes, three tablespoons of tomato puree, some of your favorite herbs such as oregano or basil. To make sauce spicier add chili flakes. Mix and boil.

◆ **Soy Sauce.** Soy sauce does have a low calorie content but it has around 900mg of sodium per spoonful. When your sodium intake is too high it can lead to hypertension, such as high blood pressure. If you have high blood pressure this could lead to other more serious health problems such as stroke and heart attack.
Another Choice: The good news is there are healthier alternatives for soy sauce that have reduced sodium.

◆ **Multigrain products.** Products that contain refined grains are much less healthy than whole grains. Refined grains lack nutritional value, and they are strongly connected with weight gain.
Another Choice: When choosing breads and pastas it is best to go with a wholegrain and wholemeal product.

◆ **Foods Containing Artificial Sweeteners.** Even though artificial sweeteners contain no calories, many of them (such as aspartame) seem to impair your body's ability to detect whether your stomach is full, triggering overeating and stronger cravings that can damage your attempts to lose weight.
Another Choice: You should instead choose natural sweeteners.

◆ **Sugary Cereals.** You are best to stay away from sugary cereals such as Cocoa Frosted Flakes that tops out at 88 percent of calories from sugar. Experts say that sugar should account for no more than 25 percent of your daily intake.

Another Choice: You should make your own homemade cereal—use steel cut oats, unsweetened coconut, almonds, dried fruit or anything else you can add that is healthy, such as topping it off with a handful of blueberries, and pouring almond milk on top.

Healthy Breakfast Recipe Collection

1. Avocado with Eggs
Total Calories: 187

Ingredients:

- half an avocado, 117 calories
- Sunny side up egg, 70 calories

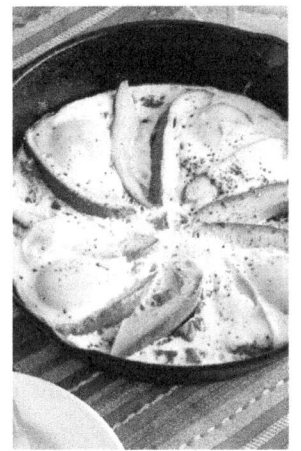

2. Egg White Omelette
Total Calories: 140

Ingredients:

- three egg whites, 51 calories
- one ounce of feta cheese, 75 calories
- two cups of baby spinach, 14 calories

3. Yogurt Smoothie
Total Calories: 240

Ingredients:

- one sliced banana, 100 calories
- half a cup of strawberries, 27 calories
- half a cup of blueberries, 42 calories
- half a container of plain Greek yogurt, 50 calories
- one teaspoon of honey, 21 calories

Directions:

Add all ingredients to blender and blend until nice and smooth.

4. Cottage Cheese with Fruit & Nuts
Total Calories: 306

Ingredients:

- one cup of cottage cheese, 220 calories
- quarter cup of banana, 33 calories
- quarter cup of blueberries, 21 calories
- tablespoon of chopped walnuts, 32 calories

5. Wheat Toast & Peanut butter
Total Calories: 210

Ingredients:

- one tablespoon of peanut butter, 90 calories
- one slice of whole wheat toast, 120 calories

6. Oatmeal
Total Calories: 262

Ingredients:

- one cup of oatmeal, 150 calories
- half a cup of blueberries, 42 calories
- half a cup of strawberries, 27 calories
- one sliced apple, 70 calories

7. Greek Yogurt
Total Calories: 100

Good breakfast especially if you are in a hurry, have 5.3 ounces of nonfat Greek yogurt, it is full of protein.

8. Low-Calorie Breakfast Burrito
Total Calories: 205

Ingredients:
- one whole wheat tortilla, 80 calories
- three scrambled egg whites, 51 calories
- one piece of turkey bacon, 30 calories
- half a slice of mozzarella cheese, 38 calories
- quarter of a tomato, 5 calories
- one tablespoon of basil, 1 calorie

Directions:

Roll the cooked egg, slice of bacon, cheese, tomato, basil up inside tortilla and enjoy!

9. Toast with Ricotta Cheese
Total Calories: 310

Ingredients:
- two slices of toasted whole grain bread, 250 calories
- two tablespoons of ricotta cheese, 51 calories
- three slices of tomato, 9 calories

Directions:

Top one slice of toast with first spreading on ricotta cheese, then add slices of tomato and top with second piece of toast and enjoy!

10. Yogurt Mix
Total Calories: 201

Ingredients:
- one container of Greek plain yogurt, 100 calories
- one cup of fresh blueberries, 80 calories
- one teaspoon of honey, 21 calories

Directions:

Mix all ingredients together in a bowl and then enjoy!

11. Apple Yogurt Cinnamon Pancakes
Total Calories: 245 yields 4 servings
Ingredients:

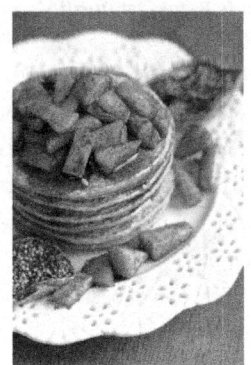

- one egg
- half a teaspoon of baking soda
- one teaspoon of baking powder
- one tablespoon of Stevia for baking
- one tablespoon of canola oil
- one cup of plain fat-free yogurt
- one teaspoon of cinnamon
- pinch of salt
- butter-flavored cooking spray
- half a cup thinly sliced apple
- one cup of almond flour

Directions:

Combine egg, oil and yogurt in blender until smooth. Sift flour, Stevia, baking powder, baking soda, cinnamon and salt together. Add yogurt mixture and blend. Prepare hot griddle with butter spray. Ladle one eighth of a cup of mixture onto griddle. Sprinkle with apples and cook until bubbles form in pancake. Flip over and cook until done.

12. Creamy Fruit-Topped Waffles
Total Calories: 281 yields 2 servings
Ingredients:

- half a cup of dry oatmeal
- one sliced banana
- one teaspoon of vanilla
- one teaspoon of cinnamon
- two tablespoons of Stevia
- three egg whites
- half a cup of non-fat cottage cheese
- two tablespoons of heavy cream
- half a cup of sliced strawberries

Directions:

Combine all ingredients in a blender except fruit and cream. Mix sliced fruit with heavy cream in separate bowl. Pour batter onto waffle maker. Once cooked, top with creamy fruit topping.

13. Egg & Spinach Cupcakes
Total Calories: 175 yields 5 servings

Ingredients:

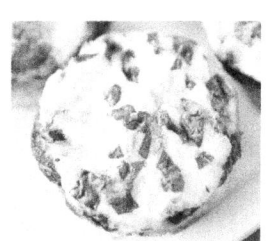

- ◆ ten ounces of frozen spinach, chopped
- ◆ one cup of low-fat mozzarella cheese, shredded
- ◆ one cup of skim ricotta cheese
- ◆ two eggs

Directions:

Preheat oven to 350° Fahrenheit. Place cupcake liners in 12-hole cupcake tin. Heat spinach in microwave until warm. Whip the eggs add spinach. Fold in the ricotta and shredded cheese. Fill each cup with egg-spinach mixture about half. Bake for 35 minutes.

14. Cheese & Chive Omelette
Total Calories: 156 yields 2 servings

Ingredients:

- ◆ one large egg
- ◆ four large egg whites
- ◆ two tablespoons of fresh chives, chopped
- ◆ one quarter cup of reduced-fat cheddar, shredded
- ◆ one tablespoon of olive oil
- ◆ one quarter of a teaspoon of sea salt

Directions:

Beat egg and egg whites in a bowl and mix in salt. Heat the olive oil in small skillet on low heat. Pour the egg mixture into skillet. Cook until edges are firm. Sprinkle cheese over it, and also sprinkle the chives over it. Fold one side over the other. Flip half-moon omelette so both sides are cooked.

Healthy Lunch Recipe Collection

1. Ground Turkey Lettuce Wrap
Total Calories: **232**
Ingredients:

- one large leaf of Boston Lettuce, 2 calories
- four ounces of lean ground turkey, cooked, 151 calories
- one teaspoon of fresh ginger, 2 calories
- one teaspoon of garlic, minced, 5 calories
- half a cup of shredded carrots, 20 calories
- one quarter of a chopped red bell pepper, 6 calories
- one teaspoon of cilantro, chopped, 1 calorie

Directions:

Cook ground turkey over medium high heat add in ginger, and garlic, mix well, cook for five minutes or until cooked through. Add turkey to lettuce leaf, top with shredded carrots and red bell pepper, and some chopped cilantro.

2. Hummus Wrap
Total Calories: **284**
Ingredients:

- half a cup of hummus, 180 calories
- one whole wheat tortilla, 80 calories
- half a cucumber, 24 calories

Directions:

Add hummus to tortilla, add the cucumber in slices and roll and enjoy!

3. Eggplant Pizza
Total Calories: 211

Ingredients:

- one eggplant, 136 calories
- tomato sauce to each slice, 4 calories
- one ounce of mozzarella, shredded, 70 calories

Directions:

Cut the eggplant into round one inch thick pieces. Add the tomato sauce then mozzarella cheese. Can eat raw or bake for 25 minutes at 325° Fahrenheit for 25 minutes or until done. Place on baking sheet sprayed with non-stick cooking spray.

4. Cucumber Sandwich
Total Calories: 143

Ingredients:

- one cucumber, 47 calories
- tablespoon of cottage cheese, 48 calories
- two slices of turkey meat, 44 calories

Directions:

Partially peel cucumber and cut in half lengthwise. Spread cream cheese over it then add turkey slices.

5. Shrimp and Asparagus
Total Calories: 246

Ingredients:

- one pound of asparagus, 90 calories
- one cup of medium sized shrimp, 150 calories
- one teaspoon of garlic, minced, 4 calories
- squeeze of lemon juice, 2 calories

Directions:

Sauteed your asparagus, add shrimp, garlic, and lemon juice, cook until shrimp have turned pink.

6. Homemade Salad
Total Calories: 254

Ingredients:

- half a head of romaine lettuce, chopped, 50 calories
- half a medium sized tomato sliced, 11 calories
- one boiled egg, 70 calories
- half a cucumber, 23 calories
- half a yellow pepper, 25 calories
- two slices of avocado, 32 calories
- dressing use one tablespoon of red wine vinegar, 3 calories
- and one teaspoon of olive oil, 40 calories

Directions:

Chop up the romaine lettuce into a bowl, add tomato slices, avocado, sliced egg, yellow bell pepper, mix red wine vinegar and olive oil in separate bowl then pour over salad and enjoy!

7. Turkey Burger
Total Calories: 236

Ingredients:

- turkey patty, 175 calories
- one leaf of romaine lettuce, 1 calorie
- slice of tomato, 4 calories
- two slices of avocado, 32 calories
- one slice of onion, 5 calories
- one tablespoon of ketchup, 19 calories

Directions:

Bake turkey patty in oven or on stove top, or grill. Add romaine lettuce on top of patty without bun, add tomato, avocado, onion, and ketchup.

8. Kale Caesar
Total Calories: 177

Ingredients:

- two cups of kale, 66 calories
- half a cup of medium sized shrimp, 60 calories
- half a medium tomato, chopped, 11 calories
- two tablespoons of fat-free Caesar dressing, 40 calories

Directions:

Add kale to large bowl, and cooked shrimp, tomato, mix and add dressing.

9. Spinach & Strawberry Salad
Total Calories: 228

Ingredients:

- two cups of baby spinach, 14 calories
- one cup of sliced strawberries, 54 calories
- one ounce of Gorgonzola cheese, 95 calories
- one tablespoon of poppy seed dressing, 65 calories

Directions:

Add spinach to large bowl, then add strawberries, and cheese, mix and top with poppy seed dressing.

10. Tomato Salad
Total Calories: 300

Ingredients:

- one medium sliced tomato, 24 calories
- five basil leaves, 1 calorie
- three slices of mozzarella cheese, 230 calories
- one teaspoon of balsamic dressing, 5 calories
- one teaspoon of olive oil, 40 calories

Directions:

Add all ingredients in a bowl and mix well and enjoy!

11. Vegetable Soup
Total Calories: 127 yields 4-6 servings

Ingredients:

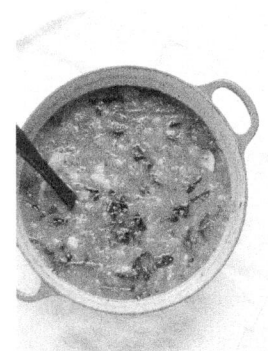

- ◆ one pound of mixed veggies
- ◆ four cups of water
- ◆ one eight ounce can of corn
- ◆ three tablespoons of vegetable bouillon
- ◆ six celery sticks, chopped
- ◆ one 28 ounce can of crushed tomatoes
- ◆ four teaspoons of Worcestershire sauce
- ◆ one teaspoon of black pepper
- ◆ one teaspoon of sea salt
- ◆ one onion, chopped

Directions:

Bring water to a boil in large pot. Add in mixed veggies, onion, corn, and celery. Stir in the vegetable bouillon. Add in crushed tomatoes, add Worcestershire sauce, black pepper and sea salt.

12. Beef Tacos
Total Calories: 483 yields 4 servings

Ingredients:

- ◆ one pound of extra lean ground beef
- ◆ eight hard taco shells
- ◆ one tablespoon of canola oil
- ◆ four ounces of Mexican cheese, shredded
- ◆ half a head of lettuce, shredded
- ◆ half a cup of non-fat sour cream
- ◆ one small onion, diced

- ◆ one tomato, diced

Directions:

- ◆ In a skillet brown beef in canola oil over medium heat on top of oven for ten minutes or so. Mix taco seasoning with ground beef and water to taste. Warm taco shells in oven at 325° Fahrenheit for 10 minutes. Spoon meat into taco shell and layer the rest of the ingredients on top of meat.

13. Crabmeat, Tomato, and Egg Salad Sandwich
Total Calories: 493 yields 4 servings

Ingredients:

- ◆ one and a half cups of cooked crabmeat
- ◆ four tablespoons of Miracle Whip salad dressing
- ◆ twelve slices of whole wheat bread
- ◆ half a cup of watercress, coarsely chopped
- ◆ one head of lettuce
- ◆ two large tomatoes thinly sliced
- ◆ small bowl of egg salad

Directions:

Smooth crabmeat add a bit of Miracle Whip to moistened it. Add to one slice of bread. Top with tomato slices and dash of salt and pepper. Place another slice of bread over top. Smooth some egg salad on the top add watercress, finish with final piece of bread.

14. Eggplant and Portobello Mushroom Melt
Total Calories: 483 yields 4 servings

Ingredients:

- ◆ one large eggplant sliced lengthwise in half inch slices
- ◆ one small Vidalia onion, sliced
- ◆ half a cup of canola oil
- ◆ four large Portobello mushroom caps
- ◆ salt and pepper to taste

- eight slices of whole wheat bread
- four leaves of lettuce
- two tablespoons of fresh thyme
- one third of a cup of parsley, chopped
- half a cup of fat-free Miracle Whip salad dressing

Directions:

Brush eggplant, onion, and mushrooms with oil. Season with salt and pepper. Grill mushrooms, onion, and eggplant slices on both sides until tender. Mix parsley, thyme and Miracle Whip. Toast or grill slices of bread. Thinly spread Miracle Whip mix on grilled bread. Arrange slices of vegetables on one side of bread. Top with lettuce leaf and another slice of bread.

Healthy Dinner Recipe Collection

1. Roasted Vegetable Lasagna
Total Calories: 429

Ingredients:

- ◆ one package of light lasagna noodles, 260 calories
- ◆ one red bell pepper, chopped, 24 calories
- ◆ one cup of squash, 20 calories
- ◆ one medium sized chopped onion, 42 calories
- ◆ one cup of tomato sauce, 70 calories
- ◆ one teaspoon of garlic, minced, 13 calories

Directions:

Cook your noodles in pot of boiling water, once they have cooked, drain and allow to cool. Chop up onion, cube squash, chop pepper, mix up in a bowl, add garlic and mix some more. In baking pan add half a cup of tomato sauce on bottom then layer with noodles, add veggies, and layer some more noodles then top with remaining tomato sauce. Bake on 325° Fahrenheit for 45 minutes or until cooked.

2. Brown Rice with Veggies
Total Calories: 374

Ingredients:

- ◆ half a cup of cooked brown rice, 100 calories
- ◆ one large scrambled egg, 70 calories
- ◆ one teaspoon of sesame oil, 40 calories
- ◆ one cup of chopped zucchini, 21 calories
- ◆ one cup of chopped carrots, 49 calories
- ◆ one medium onion, chopped, 42 calories
- ◆ one cup of broccoli, chopped, 31 calories

Directions:

Once your rice is cooked mix in all the other ingredients and enjoy!

3. Brown Rice Chicken Stir Fry
Total Calories: 465

Ingredients:

- ◆ half a cup of brown rice, cooked, 100 calories
- ◆ one pound of chicken cut into one inch cubes, 150 calories
- ◆ one medium onion, chopped, calories 42
- ◆ one cup of mushrooms, chopped, 21 calories
- ◆ one green pepper, chopped, calories 24

Directions:

Cook veggies and chicken in a skillet with some olive oil (two tablespoons 119 calories), Add tablespoon of low-sodium soy sauce (9 calories) for taste. Cook over medium heat until veggies are softened and chicken is cooked through—about 20 minutes.

4. Cabbage Soup
Total Calories: 377

Ingredients:

- ◆ one small head of cabbage, 165 calories
- ◆ one medium onion, chopped, 42 calories
- ◆ one cup of chicken broth, 32 calories
- ◆ one cup of tomato juice, 41 calories
- ◆ one cup of fresh beans, chopped, 30 calories
- ◆ one cup of chopped celery, 16 calories
- ◆ one cup of carrots, chopped, 51 calories

Directions:

Put all of the ingredients into a crock pot and cook for two hours on high.

5. Veggies with Quinoa
Total Calories: 437

Ingredients:

- One cup of cooked quinoa, 223 calories
- one cup of sweet potatoes, chopped, calories 160
- one cup of mushrooms, chopped, calories 21
- one cup of kale, shredded, 33 calories

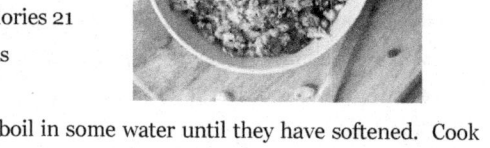

Directions:

Cook all the veggies in a pot together and boil in some water until they have softened. Cook Quinoa separately in another pot. Mix all in one big pot once they are cooked.

6. Chicken & Artichokes
Total Calories: 339

Ingredients:

- one cup of tomatoes, chopped, 32 calories
- half a cup of water and one can of cooked artichokes, 150 calories
- one pound of boneless, skinless, chicken breast, 150 calories
- half a cup of white wine vinegar, 7 calories
- salt and pepper to taste

Directions:

Cook chicken breast on top of stove in skillet with white wine vinegar over medium high heat for about ten minutes or until chicken is cooked through. Add water, artichokes, and tomatoes and mix. Cook for an additional ten minutes and enjoy!

7. Baked Chicken and Greens
Total Calories: 378

Ingredients:

- one tablespoon of olive oil, 119 calories

- ◆ one whole squeezed lemon, 10 calories
- ◆ one cup of Brussels sprouts, 38 calories
- ◆ two cups of fresh green beans, 61 calories
- ◆ one boneless, skinless, chicken breast, 150 calories

Directions:

Mix all ingredients with lemon juice. Add one tablespoon of olive oil to bottom of baking pan. Cook all ingredients in baking pan in oven at 400° Fahrenheit for 45 minutes.

8. Zesty Shrimp with Potato & Asparagus
Total Calories: 285

Ingredients:

- ◆ one medium boiled potato, 140 calories
- ◆ half a pound of asparagus, steamed, 45 calories
- ◆ one teaspoon of garlic, minced 5 calories
- ◆ half a squeeze of fresh lemon juice, 6 calories
- ◆ one tablespoon of parsley, fresh, 1 calorie
- ◆ one dozen medium shrimp, 48 calories
- ◆ one tablespoon of olive oil, 40 calories

Directions:

Heat olive oil in skillet on top of stove over medium heat. Once oil is hot add in the dozen shrimp, parsley, garlic, lemon juice. For sides use the asparagus and boiled potato.

9. Chinese Chicken Stir Fry
Total Calories: 198

Ingredients:

- ◆ one ounce of carrots, chopped, 10 calories
- ◆ one ounce of cauliflower, chopped, 7 calories
- ◆ one ounce of broccoli, chopped, 9 calories
- ◆ one ounce of snow peas, 12 calories
- ◆ one tablespoon of soy sauce, 9 calories

- ◆ one tablespoon of honey, 64 calories
- ◆ one boneless, skinless, chicken breast
- ◆ one teaspoon of sesame seeds, 17 calories

Directions:

Cut the chicken into cubes, cook over medium heat with honey, soy sauce, and sesame seeds. Make veggies by steaming them and add as a side to dish.

10. Roasted Pork & Brussels Sprouts
Total Calories: 282

Ingredients:

- ◆ two cups of Brussels sprouts, 76 calories
- ◆ one teaspoon of olive oil, 40 calories
- ◆ one 3.5 ounce fillet of boneless pork loin, 166 calories

Directions:

In a roasting pan place the pork on a rack and below the roasting pan Brussels sprouts spread with olive oil. Add salt and pepper to taste and bake for 45 minutes at 325° Fahrenheit or until done.

11. Tuna Casserole
Total Calories: 278 yields 4 servings

Ingredients:

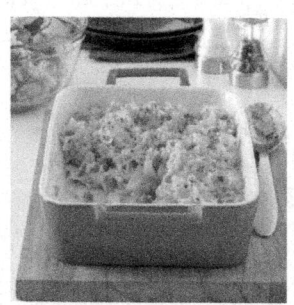

- ◆ one can of cream of chicken soup, low-sodium
- ◆ two cups of whole wheat macaroni noodles
- ◆ ten ounces of frozen cut green beans
- ◆ one six ounce can of tuna, drained
- ◆ half a cup of fat-free milk
- ◆ one quarter of a teaspoon of fresh ground pepper
- ◆ five tablespoons of breadcrumbs

Directions:

Mix soup and milk in a bowl. In another bowl mix noodles, tuna, pepper, add soup and milk mix and gently fold. Put into baking dish and cover with foil. Bake for 25 minutes then uncover and put breadcrumbs on top and bake until breadcrumbs are browned.

12. Beef Stroganoff
Total Calories: 488 yields 4 servings

Ingredients:

◆ one large onion, finely chopped
◆ one quarter cup of canola oil
◆ one teaspoon of garlic, minced
◆ one pound of lean flank steak
◆ two cups of mushrooms, sliced
◆ one tablespoon corn starch
◆ two tablespoons of cooking sherry
◆ one cup of beef broth, low-sodium
◆ one cup of fat-free sour cream
◆ two cups of cooked wide noodles
◆ half a cup of parsley, finely chopped
◆ salt and pepper to taste

Directions:

Thinly slice steak. Saute onions over medium heat, add the steak in canola oil, then add mushrooms and garlic, heat until tender. Mix cornstarch, sherry and broth in small bowl. Make a paste, pour it into meat mixture and let simmer for five minutes, add salt and pepper, and sour cream. Pour over hot noodles and garnish with parsley.

13. Beef and Vegetable Cheese Casserole
Total Calories: 398 yields 4 servings

Ingredients:

◆ one medium onion, chopped
◆ two tablespoons of canola oil
◆ one pound of lean ground beef

- one nine-ounce bag of frozen mixed vegetables
- half a cup of non-fat sour cream
- eight ounces of cheddar cheese, low-fat

Directions:

Heat the oil in a skillet and brown onions, add ground beef. Microwave mixed vegetables until thawed. Drain fat from fully browned meat. Add vegetables and non-fat sour cream to the skillet and mix well. Pour into casserole dish and sprinkle with cheese.

14. Salmon Loaf
Total Calories: 196 yields 8 servings
Ingredients:

- half cup of shallots, chopped
- half a cup of light Ritz crackers, crushed
- two tablespoons of olive oil
- half a cup of fat-free milk
- one egg, beaten
- four teaspoons of lemon juice
- one fourteen ounce can of salmon

Directions:

Preheat your oven to 350° Fahrenheit. Heat the olive oil in a skillet over medium heat. Sauté the shallots until tender. In a large bowl, mix cracker crumbs, milk, egg, shallots, and lemon juice. Beat well. Add the salmon to the bowl and mix well. Lightly spray a baking pan. Place salmon mixture in the baking pan and bake for one hour or until brown.

Healthy Snacks/Desserts Collection

1. Watermelon Slushie with Boba Recipe
Total Calories: 198

Ingredients:

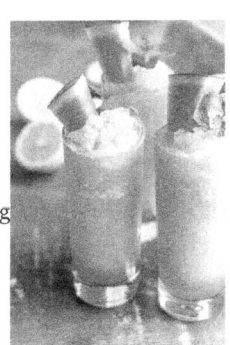

- ◆ two tablespoons of dried boba tapioca pearls
- ◆ two tablespoons of cold coconut water or sparkling water
- ◆ one quarter of a cup of frozen pineapple chunks
- ◆ 12 fresh mint leaves
- ◆ one teaspoon of Stevia
- ◆ juice one lime
- ◆ two cups of seedless watermelon

Directions:

Bring a cup of water to boil, add boba, stirring until it begins to float. Reduce heat to simmer until it is tender, about 15 minutes. Remove from heat and cover and let sit for 15 minutes. Rinse under cold water and drain, set aside. Combine pineapple, coconut or water, mint in blender until pureed. Pour into bottom of drinking glass. Rinse blender then add frozen watermelon, lime juice blend until it is like a slushy. Stir in the boba and gently spoon watermelon slushy on top of the pineapple mix.

2. Raw Almonds & Dried Apricots
Total Calories: 200

Ingredients:

- ◆ one ounce of almonds (around 22 nuts)
- ◆ three dried apricots

3. Fig & Walnut Energy Bars
Total Calories: 200 per bar

Ingredients:

- ◆ one and a half cups of walnuts, chopped
- ◆ one teaspoon of pure vanilla extract
- ◆ one large egg
- ◆ one cup of dried apricots, chopped
- ◆ one cup of dried Turkish figs, quartered
- ◆ one third of a cup of light brown sugar
- ◆ half a cup of dried cranberries
- ◆ half a teaspoon of cinnamon
- ◆ one quarter of a teaspoon of sea salt
- ◆ one eighth of a teaspoon of baking powder
- ◆ one third of a cup of whole-grain flour

Directions:

Preheat your oven to 325° Fahrenheit and line an 8×8-inch baking pan with parchment paper, across the bottom and on both sides. Toast walnuts in oven for 10 minutes. Remove from oven and set aside. In food processor blend, baking soda, flour, sugar, cinnamon, salt and half of each dried fruit amount. Transfer to large bowl and mix in the walnuts and the rest of dried fruit with your hands. Whisk the egg and vanilla together, then add to fruit mixture. Blend well then pack down with fingers into pan and bake for 35-40 minutes. Remove from oven and transfer to a wire rack lifting out by parchment paper and set on rack and allow to cool. Then cut into 12 pieces and store in air tight container.

4. Pumpkin Muffins
Total Calories: 124, yields 18 servings
Ingredients:

- ◆ two and a half cups of almond flour
- ◆ half a cup of Stevia for baking
- ◆ one tablespoon of baking powder
- ◆ one teaspoon of ground cinnamon
- ◆ half a teaspoon ground nutmeg
- ◆ half a teaspoon of ground ginger
- ◆ one quarter of a teaspoon of salt

- one cup of plain canned pumpkin pie filling
- two eggs
- three quarter cup of fat-free milk
- six tablespoons of melted butter

Directions:

Preheat your oven to 400° Fahrenheit. Spray muffin tin with a light cooking spray. Mix flour, Stevia, baking powder, nutmeg, cinnamon, ginger and salt in large bowl. Stir pumpkin filling, milk, eggs, and melted butter. Mix until all ingredients are well moistened. Spoon into muffin tin, each two thirds full. Bake for 20 minutes until muffin tops are golden brown.

5. Stuffed Cucumbers
Total Calories: 75, yields 4 servings

Ingredients:

- two large cucumbers
- three ounces of low-fat cream cheese
- one tablespoon low-fat blue cheese
- one teaspoon of onion, minced
- one teaspoon of parsley, dried
- one teaspoon of dill, fresh

Directions:

Create strips in the cucumber by using a vegetable peeler, about one quarter of an inch apart, lengthwise. Cut the ends off the cucumbers. Scoop out seeds and pulp from cucumbers, use a melon baller. Mix cream cheese, blue cheese, dill, parsley, and onion in small bowl. Place mixture inside the hollowed cucumbers using a pastry bag with a star tip. Cover with plastic and refrigerate for at least an hour. Cut into one inch circles and serve.

6. Stuffed Creamy Mushrooms
Total Calories: 202, yields 4-6 servings

Ingredients:

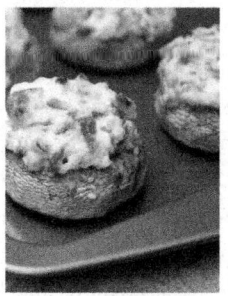

- ◆ one 16-ounce package of reduced-fat pork sausage
- ◆ juice of one lemon
- ◆ one 8-ounce package of reduced-fat cream cheese
- ◆ half a minced green pepper
- ◆ half an onion, minced
- ◆ 20-25 whole mushrooms, with stems removed

Directions:

Preheat your oven to 300° Fahrenheit. Brown sausage in skillet over medium heat on top of oven. Add onion and pepper. Cook and remove from heat, drain the fat. Mix cream cheese with lemon juice and cooled sausage mixture. Stuff each mushroom with mixture. Place on baking sheet and bake for 20 minutes.

7. Frozen Yogurt Pie
Total Calories: 186, yields 10 servings

Ingredients:

- ◆ two 8-ounce containers of nonfat vanilla yogurt
- ◆ one 16-ounce package frozen strawberries, defrosted
- ◆ one 8-ounce container of low-fat or nonfat frozen whipped topping
- ◆ one two-ounce package of strawberry gelatin
- ◆ one 9 inch pre-baked pie shell

Directions:

Mix the strawberries and yogurt in a blender and blend until creamy with small chunks of strawberries. Mix the whipped topping and gelatin in large bowl. Mix in the strawberry mixture. Pour mixture into pastry shell and freeze.

8. Oatmeal Cookies
Total Calories: 218, yields 24 cookies

Ingredients:

- one cup of Stevia for baking
- one quarter cup of butter, softened
- two eggs
- three quarter of a cup of unsweetened applesauce
- one teaspoon vanilla
- two cups of coconut flour
- half a teaspoon of baking soda
- one quarter of a teaspoon of salt
- one cup uncooked oats

Directions:

Preheat your oven to 375° Fahrenheit. Prepare baking sheets with light cooking spray and set aside. Beat the butter and Stevia in large bowl with hand mixer. Add the eggs, applesauce, and vanilla, mixing well. Combine baking soda, flour and salt in another bowl. Add the flour mix to the sugar mix and beat well. Stir in the oats, mix well. Drop the dough into mounds on baking sheets, about two inches apart. Bake for 15 minutes or until the cookies are golden.

9. Ginger Cookies
Total Calories: 138, yields 20 cookies
Ingredients:

- one and one quarter of a cup of coconut flour
- two teaspoons of ground ginger
- three tablespoons of butter, melted
- one egg white, lightly beaten
- one quarter of a cup of unsweetened applesauce
- one quarter of a cup of molasses
- one quarter of a teaspoon of vanilla
- one quarter of a cup of brown Splenda

Directions:

Sift flour and ginger in a large bowl, then stir in the Splenda. Mix the vanilla, molasses, butter, applesauce, and egg white in a bowl. Add wet ingredients to the dry ingredients and blend well. Place dough in freezer until firm. Preheat your oven to 350° Fahrenheit. Shape firm balls and drop onto baking sheet that has been sprayed with light no-stick cooking spray.

Bake for 12 minutes and let cool.

10. Light Mango Fluff
Total Calories: 148, yields 12 servings
Ingredients:

- four egg whites
- one cup of Stevia
- one tablespoon of lemon juice
- one cup of heavy whipping cream
- two tablespoons of powdered sugar
- one teaspoon of vanilla
- one cup of flaked coconut
- 7.5 ounces of frozen mangoes, thawed

Directions:

Put egg whites in large bowl, let stand for 30 minutes. Add Stevia, lemon juice, and mangoes. Beat with hand mixer until combined, then beat for 15 minutes on high speed, until it is thick. Beat cream with powdered sugar in another bowl with vanilla. Fold into meringue with coconut. Rinse out 10-inch ring mold, pour coconut mixture into mold cover and freeze until firm. To unmold, rinse kitchen towel under hot water and wring out. Put mold on plate, drape towel over mold for 15 seconds to loosen dessert, let stand at room temperature for 15 then slice and serve.

11. Lemon Pie
Total Calories: 155, yields 12 servings
Ingredients:

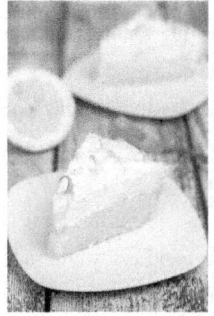

- half a cup of egg beaters
- zest and juice of two lemons
- four egg whites
- four cups of light cool whip
- five and a half ounces of vanilla wafer cookies

◆ half a cup of sugar (or you can use Stevia for baking to replace it)

Directions:

Squeeze lemons to get half a cup of juice. In a double boiler, cook the Egg Beaters, sugar, and lemon juice over simmering water until it gets thick. Remove from heat and stir in the lemon zest. Pour entire mixture into bowl and stick in refrigerator until it is cold. Whip the egg whites to form peaks. Mix about one third of the egg whites into the cold lemon mixture. Fold the rest of the egg whites and the Cool Whip topping until well blended. Crush the vanilla wafers in a freezer bag. Line two pie tins with vanilla wafer crumbs. Saving some to sprinkle over the top of pies. Fill the pie tins with the lemon mixture. Sprinkle top with Cool Whip topping and remaining wafers. Place pies in freezer until firm. Remove from freezer 10 minutes before serving

12. Apple Pie
Total Calories: 285, yields 10 servings

Ingredients:

- two cups of all-purpose flour, divided
- six tablespoons of ice water
- seven tablespoons of vegetable shortening
- two tablespoons of powdered sugar
- one teaspoon of apple-cider vinegar
- one tablespoon of sugar
- one egg white
- one teaspoon of salt
- one teaspoon of nutmeg
- one teaspoon of cinnamon
- three tablespoons of all-purpose flour
- two third cup of sugar
- one tablespoon of lemon juice
- eight cups of Granny Smith apples, peeled, and thinly sliced

Directions:

Combine half a cup of flour, ice water and vinegar, stir until well blended. Mix in remaining one and a half cups of flour, powdered sugar, and half a teaspoon of salt in bowl. Mix in shortening with two knives until the mixture is similar to coarse meal. Divide the dough in half. Gently press each half into a four inch circle on two sheets of overlapping heavy-duty plastic wrap; cover with two additional sheets of overlapping plastic wrap. Roll one dough half, still covered, into a twelve inch circle. Repeat with other half. Chill dough for 10 minutes. Prepare filling by combining the apples and lemon juice in large bowl. Mix two thirds of a cup of sugar, three tablespoons of flour, cinnamon, nutmeg, and one eighth teaspoon of salt in a bowl.

Sprinkle sugar mixture over apples and toss and coat well. Lightly spray pie plates with cooking spray. Remove top sheets of plastic wrap from 12" dough circle. Fit dough, plastic wrap side up, into pie plate, allowing dough to extend over edge. Remove the remaining plastic wrap. Spoon filling into dough; brush edges of dough lightly with water. Remove top two sheets of plastic wrap from the remaining dough circle; place, plastic wrap side up, on top of filled pie plate. Remove remaining plastic wrap. Press edges of dough together. Fold edges under. Cut several slits on top of pastry using sharp knife. Brush top and edges of pie with egg white; sprinkle with one tablespoon of sugar. Bake for 40 minutes or until top is golden brown. Chill well before you serve.

13. Crisp Cookies
Total Calories: 118, yields 48 cookies
Ingredients:
- ◆ one quarter of a cup of coconut oil
- ◆ three quarter of a cup of butter, softened
- ◆ one cup of brown sugar
- ◆ one cup of sugar
- ◆ two eggs
- ◆ one teaspoon of baking soda
- ◆ two teaspoons of vanilla
- ◆ half a teaspoon of salt
- ◆ one cup of cashews, finely chopped
- ◆ two and one quarter cups of almond flour

Directions:

In a large bowl beat butter, coconut oil, until well blended. Add brown sugar, and sugar; beat until fluffy, add eggs and vanilla and mix well. Stir in the flour, baking soda, and salt. Shape the dough into three long rolls, about one and a half inches in diameter. Roll the cookie rolls in the chopped cashews, gently pressing nuts into dough to adhere. Wrap well in wax paper, then put rolls into plastic food-storage bags. Chill for at least 24 hours. Preheat oven to 375° Fahrenheit. Cut the dough into slices about one quarter inch thick and place on ungreased baking sheets. Bake for eight minutes or until cookies are very light golden brown. Cool on cookie sheets for three minutes, then remove to wire racks to cool.

14. Apple & Oats Crisp
Total Calories: 157, yields 6 servings

Ingredients:

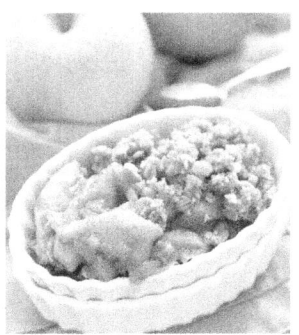

- ◆ one tablespoon of lemon juice
- ◆ four Granny Smith apples, peeled, and sliced
- ◆ three tablespoons of sugar
- ◆ one cup of uncooked oats
- ◆ two tablespoons Splenda brown sugar
- ◆ two tablespoons of butter
- ◆ one teaspoon of ground cinnamon

Directions:

Preheat your oven to 350° Fahrenheit. Combine apples, lemon juice, and sugar in large bowl, tossing and mixing. Place this apple mixture on the bottom of a nine inch pie plate. In another bowl mix the oats, Splenda brown sugar, butter, and cinnamon with your fingers to make sure the mixture is crumbly. Sprinkle the crumb mixture over apple mixture. Bake for 50 minutes or until bubbly.

14-Day Meal Planner

It is vital that you remember to keep yourself hydrated and drink plenty of water 7-8 glasses a day would be a healthy start.

Day 1	Breakfast: Avocado with Eggs Total Calories: 187 Lunch: Eggplant Pizza Total Calories: 211 Dinner: Chinese Chicken Stir Fry Total Calories: 198 Snack/Dessert: Watermelon Slushie with Boba Recipe Total Calories: 198
Day 2	Breakfast: Yogurt Mix Total Calories: 201 Lunch: Tomato Salad Total Calories: 300 Dinner: Toast with Ricotta Cheese Total Calories: 310 Snack/Dessert Spinach & Strawberry Salad Total Calories: 228

Day 3	**Breakfast:**
	Low-Calories Breakfast Burrito
	Total Calories: 205
	Lunch:
	Kale Caesar
	Total Calories: 177
	Dinner:
	Roasted Pork & Brussels Sprouts
	Total Calories: 282
	Snack/Dessert
	Raw Almonds & Dried Apricots
	Total Calories: 200
Day 4	**Breakfast:**
	Greek Yogurt
	Total Calories: 100
	Lunch:
	Kale Caesar
	Total Calories: 177
	Dinner:
	Zesty Shrimp with Potato & Asparagus
	Total Calories: 285
	Snack/Dessert
	Light Mango Fluff
	Total Calories: 148
Day 5	**Breakfast:**
	Toast with Ricotta Cheese
	Total Calories: 310
	Lunch:
	Cucumber Salad
	Total Calories: 143
	Dinner:
	Baked Chicken Greens

	Total Calories: 378
	Snack/Dessert
	Ginger Cookies
	Total Calories: 138
Day 6	**Breakfast:**
	Egg White Omelette
	Total Calories: 140
	Lunch:
	Homemade salad
	Total Calories: 284
	Dinner:
	Chicken & Artichokes
	Total Calories: 339
	Snack/Dessert
	Fig & Walnut Energy Bars
	Total Calories: 200
Day 7	**Breakfast:**
	Yogurt Smoothie
	Total Calories: 240
	Lunch:
	Hummus Wrap
	Total Calories: 284
	Dinner:
	Veggies & Quinoa
	Total Calories: 437
	Snack/Dessert
	Pumpkin Muffin
	Total Calories: 124

Day 8	**Breakfast:**
	Cottage Cheese with Fruit & Nuts
	Total Calories: 306
	Lunch:
	Eggplant Pizza
	Total Calories: 211
	Dinner:
	Roasted Vegetable Lasagna
	Total Calories: 429
	Snack/Dessert
	Stuffed Cucumbers
	Total Calories: 75
Day 9	**Breakfast:**
	Wheat Toast & Peanut Butter
	Total Calories: 210
	Lunch:
	Shrimp & Asparagus
	Total Calories: 246
	Dinner:
	Brown Rice Chicken Stir Fry
	Total Calories: 465
	Snack/Dessert
	Frozen Yogurt Pie
	Total Calories: 186

Day 10	**Breakfast:**
	Oatmeal
	Total Calories: 262
	Lunch:
	Ground Turkey Lettuce Wrap
	Total Calories: 232
	Dinner:
	Brown rice with Veggies
	Total Calories: 374
	Snack/Dessert
	Oatmeal Cookies
	Total Calories: 218
Day 11	**Breakfast:**
	Apple Yogurt Cinnamon Pancakes
	Total Calories: 245
	Lunch:
	Vegetable Soup
	Total Calories: 127
	Dinner:
	Tuna Casserole
	Total Casserole: 278
	Snack/Dessert
	Lemon Pie
	Total Calories: 155
Day 12	**Breakfast:**
	Creamy Fruit-Topped Waffles
	Total Calories: 281
	Lunch:
	Beef Tacos
	Total Calories: 483
	Dinner:
	Beef Stroganoff
	Total Calories: 488

	Snack/Dessert Apple Pie Total Calories: 285
Day 13	**Breakfast:** Egg & Spinach Cupcakes Total Calories: 175 **Lunch:** Crabmeat, Tomato and Egg salad sandwich Total Calories: 493 **Dinner:** Beef, Vegetable and Cheese Casserole Total Calories: 398 **Snack/Dessert** Crisp Cookies Total Calories: 118
Day 14 *Cheat Day-Congratulations For Completing Your First Two-weeks of Your Diet Plan, Celebrate by Having a Treat of Your Choice! Give Yourself a Cheat Day 1-2 a month!*	**Breakfast:** Cheese & Chive Omelette Total Calories: 156 **Lunch:** Eggplant & Portobello Mushroom Melt Total Calories: 483 **Dinner:** Salmon Loaf Total Calories: 196 **Snack/Dessert** Apple Crisp Total Calories: 157

Part 2. Maximize Your Weight Loss Results with Exercise!

In order to maximize your weight loss results adding some cardiovascular exercise to your routine will help to accelerate fat loss by burning calories, thereby increasing your metabolism. When you add cardio exercise to your routine it will increase heart, lungs, and muscle functions. You can increase your cardio or aerobic activity in various ways, such as walking, swimming, jogging, running, biking or rowing, Basically it is an activity that involves your heart, lungs and muscles get a workout. When you elevate your heart and lung rate, you will burn more energy than at rest. More energy equals more calories. When you combine proper cardio and proper nutrition, you have a dynamic duo that slices away the pounds.

You are going to embark on a journey that will involve enhancing both your mind and body. You are going to work towards getting rid of unwanted weight from trouble spot areas and toning up while getting healthier by the day. Setting up a routine for yourself that you have some regularity is important so that you do not slack off and drop exercising all together.

When you burn off more calories than you consume, this will trigger the burning of your fat stores. The American College Sports Medicine recommends that accumulating 250 to 300 minutes per week of moderate intensity exercise for weight loss and prevention of weight gain. When you develop an excellent routine you will be empowering yourself. Losing weight is going to be very rewarding and satisfying work. Once you start to see the results, this will give you a positive boost to continue to workout and eat properly. You may even find that it will become almost like an addiction. It will become a habit—a good habit—one that you do not want to break.

Plan
The most important aspect of an effective exercise plan is consistency. If you are willing to

put in the time every day, your body is going to burn calories and the weight is going to drop off. There is no reason that you should become stressed about a workout plan—make sure that it is one that is realistic—if not you will set yourself up for failure and disappointment. Do give yourself empty promises. A beginner should be able to burn 10 to 11 calories in a few minutes of working out. So if you are working out in a timeframe of 45 minutes you should burn around 500 calories.

The great equalizer is time, when you add more time to your workout, along with additional resistance; you will strengthen your heart, build your muscles, making them more efficient fuel burners. Your endurance and energy will be increased. Your heart will become stronger, your muscles with strengthen, your lungs will expand, and you will become more physically fit as a result.

What you choose as your cardio routine is of course your personal choice, but I will offer some suggestions in this chapter that you may find to your liking. The first is and elliptical workout. When using an elliptical piece of machinery it will give you a low-impact workout. This means that it will not cause unusual pounding to your joints, knees, hips, lower back, and neck.

Warm Up.
Before you start any exercise plan you must give your body a chance to warm up—it is not unlike a machine that you first need to warm its motor up before it can operate properly. Your body needs to be able to warm up before the real task begins. Once you have warmed up the muscles, they will be able to perform better and utilize energy better. If you do not warm up you run a higher risk of cramping up, having a sprain or straining some ligament. This is due to the fact that your body is not used to the stress that you are suddenly putting on it. Before you begin exercising do at least three of the warm up exercises below for at least 3-5 minutes.

1. Spot Jogging. Stand straight with your feet spread apart. Bend your arms at the elbows and hold your palms close to your chest. Jog on the spot by lifting your feet alternately, back to back. Do not lift your feet too high. Do this for 3-5 minutes. You will begin to feel the warmth surging into your muscles. This is going to increase your blood flow to the muscles of your legs, arms and back. It will set the tone for more strenuous exercises.

2. Toe Touches. Stand with your feet hip-width apart. Bend forward as if stopping and try and touch your toes. Hold this position for a few seconds. Repeat for ten counts. This will help prevent your back from taking a sudden shock while exercising.

3. Joint Rotations. This is a great exercise that can help prevent joint injuries. Stand straight and lift your right ankle. Rotate your foot 360°. Do this for each foot for 10 counts forward and backward. Pull feet apart and rotate hips for ten counts in either clockwise and anti-clockwise directions. Also do the same for your wrists and neck.

4. Semi-Squats. Stand straight with your feet apart. Raise and outstretch your hands at the shoulder level, with your palms facing the floor and fingers pointing forward. Bend your knees and lower your hips by a foot. Come back up after five seconds. Repeat for ten counts. This warm up will help initiate your back, glutes, thighs and abdominal muscles.

5. Shoulder Shrugs & Rolls. Stand straight with your feet together. Place your arms at your sides. Roll both of your shoulders together, forwards, and backwards alternately. Roll in both directions for 10 counts each. Follow with shrugs. Pull your shoulders upwards as you do when you shrug. Hold for a second or two. Pull them back down to neutral. Repeat this for ten counts.

6. Heel Digs. Stand with your feet slightly apart and slide the right heel ahead. Place the right foot ahead roughly a foot, on the heel. Pull back the right foot and do the same with the left heel. Alternate both feet for 60 digs. Try and accomplish 60 digs within a minute for a real stretch of thighs, calves and feet. This is going to help you from getting sprained muscles or torn ligaments.

Stretches.
To finish up your warm up it is good to end it with a few stretches. It is important that you release all the tension that the exercise builds in your muscles. When stretching it will not only release the tensed feeling that you experience after a workout, but also get rid of any mild pain that you might be experiencing. The stretches will have you feeling like you did before doing any exercise, instead of feeling drained.

Stretch your arms and legs ahead of you while sitting on the floor. Stretch as much as you can. Or lie flat on your back, stretch your arms overhead and legs below and feel your abdominal and back muscles being stretched out. A third alternative is to bend your leg behind at the knee, while standing and pulling your toes with the same side hand. This will stretch out the arms as well as the legs. Do this for a few repetitions or in between two exercise sets for better performance. Now that you have completed your warm up session you are ready to jump into your exercise routine of choice! Below are some choices for you to check out.

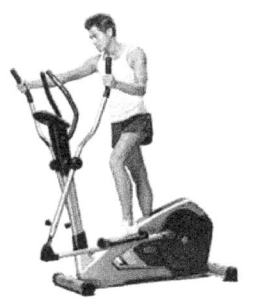

Elliptical Workout
It offers you a full body workout for your legs, glutes abdomen, lower back, shoulders, arms and chest. There is an assortment of preset and manual settings, along with the ability to pedal backward, which will target your hamstrings and glutes. Pedaling forward works the quads. When you use elliptical machines to workout on they mimic the natural movements of thighs, knees, and ankle joints like walking or jogging.

The benefit is this equipment doesn't affect your joints. There is a smooth movement. Most models of elliptical machines let you reverse pedal, which will provide you with a more versatile workout for calf and hamstring muscles. The machines that offer moving handrails keep your arms and upper body moving, while providing and overall full body workout. This will quickly elevate your heart rate, allowing you to experience a wonderful cardiovascular workout. In a 60 minute workout you will be able to burn around 600 to 800 calories. It is a good idea to get acquainted with the machine that you are going to workout on. Learn about the movements it offers, it computer programs, and its capabilities. If you are going to be going to a fitness center or club, ask a trainer to give you a demonstration of how the machine works that you are interested in using. If you have a machine at home check out the manufacture's website for instructions, tutorials, and workouts.

You should always enter your age and weight into the machine. This will help the machine to better regulate the program to maximize your results based on your criteria. Make the most of your workout and remember to vary the resistance levels each session. Increasing the resistance improves your overall cardio workout. Stand upright and use good posture, don't slouch. Slouching reduces the workload on your legs. Make sure that when you are using the machine to keep your movements fluid and in control.

You do not need to do the same routine day in and day out, you can vary your workout program. To prevent your workout from becoming boring you need to vary your routine so that you will keep training your muscles and burning away the fat. You can add spurts of speed into your workout to change things up. This can really be a good calorie burner. Pull and push the handrails with vigor to maximize your upper body workout. Focus on your workout.

Make sure that you keep yourself hydrated, keeping a bottle of water with you is always a good idea. Even though using the elliptical machine will give you an excellent full-body workout that can melt fat away, it is still a good idea to incorporate other exercises into your workout routine. It will help to prevent your workout routine from becoming boring. Here are some additional choices of exercises to do at home:

Isometric Wall Squats.
Place your back against a wall, and bend your knees, working to a 90-degree sitting position, holding the position for as long as you can. This is a great exercise to do while watching TV. This exercise will help to tone your quads.

Sit-ups.
Doing some sit-ups will help to strengthen your core.

Push-ups and Isometric Holds.
These will help to strengthen you arms, back, shoulders, and abdomen. An isometric hold is a 90-degree push-up held for an extended count.

1. Lie down with your tummy facing the floor, arms outstretched, palms flat on the floor and fingers facing ahead and legs resting on the toes.

2. Keep your head and spine aligned in a straight line, with your feet together and toes tucked and resting on the floor.

3. Phase down—bending gradually at the elbows, lower yourself towards the floor, keeping the torso and back rigid. Exhale as you go down. Try to touch your chin to the mat below. Hold this position for 15 seconds.

4. Phase-up pressing the arms, straighten out the elbows, inhaling deeply. Maintain stability and rigidity of your back and torso.

5. Repeat exercise for ten counts.

Doggy Push-ups.
This exercise will help to target your arms, legs and buttocks.

1. Start with being on all-fours like a dog, with your hands and fingers facing north. Step back, step by step, until you are in a push-up position. Reposition your feet so as to allow complete

extension of your body. Prevent your ribcage from sagging towards the floor.

2. Phase-up as you exhale, keeping your head in line with your spine, shift your weight back so the resulting position is an inverted V. Without lifting your head, press your heels on the floor. Avoid bending your knees. Hold this position for 15 seconds.

3. Phase-down by inhaling as you return to the original push-up dog position, keeping your body aligned. Repeat for ten counts.

Bent Knee Push-ups.

This exercise targets your arms, chest, and shoulders.

1. Start in the push-up position, with your arms outstretched below your shoulders, torso and back rigidly aligned with your head, tummy facing the floor and toes tucked below the feet. Rest your knees on the floor.

2. Phase-down by holding your torso and back aligned with your head, bend your elbows and lower yourself towards the floor without bending your hips. Lower yourself until your chin touches the floor. Exhale as you go down. Hold this position for 15 seconds.

3. Phase-up by pressing your palms, push your body up, straightening out your elbows. Do not let your back, tummy or hips sag. Repeat for ten counts.

Chin-ups and Pull-ups.

Doing these exercises at least once a week are great for shoulders, upper back, triceps, biceps workout. If you want to add more muscle, incorporating strength training and other isometric exercises is a good choice.

Walking.

If you are someone that has been away from doing any kind of exercise for quite sometimes walking is a low-impact form of exercise to get you started on the road to getting back into shape. If you have a dog this is a great way to get you and your dog some much needed exercise. He will certainly be a good supporter in getting you up and out the door for a daily walk I am sure. My own dog always starts to let me know it is time for a walk, in the afternoons—as that is when we go for our walks—its like she has a built-in clock. But I know there has been days that if it weren't for my dog I would have missed going for walks. You may want to find yourself a walk-buddy or you may enjoy it as being your one-on-one time with yourself. A good brisk 15-20 minutes walk a day will have you feeling more energized in no-time.

Chest Stretch.

Your chest will be targeted in this exercise.

1. Stand with your feet flat on the floor, two-feet apart, toes facing ahead and arms on either side. Do not allow your back or tummy to sag. Keep your head and back aligned during this exercise.

2. Exhale and lift your chest outwards and upwards. Rotate your shoulders outwards as you do this, pulling your shoulder blades together behind you. Hold this position for 15 seconds. Repeat 10 times.

Straight Lunge.

Your buttocks, hips, thighs and abs will be targeted in this exercise.

1. Stand with your feet joined and pull your shoulders up square. To keep your spine aligned, straight and erect, use your abdominal muscles. Do not slouch your back, allow your arms to hang loosely at your sides.

2. Slowly lift your left foot off the floor and then place it about two-feet ahead. Plant your foot firmly on the floor. Make sure to get your balance and try not to wobble. Slowly shift your weight unto your left foot. Avoid tilting and swaying your upper body forwards towards foot.

3. While you are doing the lunge forward, keep your focus on the movement downward. Continue to lower your lower body until your extended thigh is parallel to the floor. Hold this position for 15 seconds.

4. Firmly push the left foot off the floor and return to the original standing position. Repeat for 10 counts. Repeat with taking the other foot forward.

Limb Raises.

Parts of your body that are targeted in this exercise are your back, buttocks, hips, and shoulders.

1. Lie flat on your tummy on the floor or mat. Keep your arms extended in front of you, with fingers pointing ahead. Your elbows and wrists should both be completely straight. Keep the legs and toes extended straight as well. Keep your head and spine aligned. Relax the neck and let your head rest on the floor.

2. Start exhaling slowly as you lift both your legs and your arms up and away from the floor—you will look like superman flying. Lift your limbs a few inches of the floor and tighten your buttock and abdominal muscles as you do that to maintain balance. Do not lift your head or arch your back. Hold this position for 10 seconds. Repeat 10 counts.

You can also find an assortment of other exercises if you go to fitness websites. Now we have covered your diet, and exercise plans-let us now take a look into preparing your self mentally in the final section of the book—Part 3.

Part 3. Preparing Yourself Mentally to Succeed with Your Diet Plan

You need to prepare yourself mentally for "D-Day" or other words the first day of your diet. You are going to be making a lot of different changes from your eating habits, to your physical activity, and your whole mental outlook on working towards achieving your weight loss goals. It is going to be very difficult when it comes to changing bad habits that you have lived with for a very long time. You have to retrain your brain to rethink it's outlook on how you live your daily life and get ready to make a new lifestyle change. You have to get yourself emotionally prepared for your challenge that lies ahead of you. Getting into a mindset where you are ready to make the change.

A good way to help prepare yourself on a psychological level is to to give yourself a specific starting date. When you give this advance notice it will serve two main purposes. First, it will allow you time to prepare yourself emotionally, and prepare to begin the journey towards releasing that skinnier version of you trapped within. You will not be caught off-guard, but instead you will be getting yourself in a mindset to prepare for your challenge that lies ahead of you. Secondly, by giving yourself that advanced noticed of a starting date it will give you some time to say goodbye to some of those fatty treats and bad habits, that you had become very attached to in your unhealthy lifestyle.

Another good thing with having a start date is to alert those around you of what your plan is, you will find other people around you can help give you added support to get you through those tough days ahead. You may even want to find a diet buddy perhaps online or in-person, where you can offer each other support and encouragement as you go through the diet plan and lifestyle change together. You will have a better chance of sticking to your diet plan if you do have some kind of support system setup. On those particularly hard days when you feel like packing it all in—contact your support to talk it through and get that extra boost you need to continue forward with your challenge.

By giving yourself at least a week to prepare mentally for your diet, you will have time to get yourself into the right frame of mind so that you will have a better chance at succeeding in your weight loss goals. Tell yourself there will be no more bad habits once your start date begins, such as overeating, and not exercising. Your start date is the day that you will have to get up off the couch and get active—no more spending your days lying on the couch—munching on too much junk food, gaining more and more weight. By doing your exercise plan, and starting to follow your meal planner—you are going to embark on a wonderful journey that will have hard times—but in the end you will reap so many benefits from this new lifestyle change!

To make the commitment more real make a point of putting your start date on your personal calendar. This will make it seem more real for you, it is right there in front of you in black and white—it is part of your future schedule. You will look forward to starting your challenge, especially when you think of how unhappy you feel being so overweight and out of shape. You are at a much higher risk level of developing all kinds of serious life threatening ailments such as suffering from a heart attack, diabetes, and stroke, when you are overweight. Just from a health perspective, you need to get your weight down to lower you chances of ending up with a serious health issue. Getting yourself into healthy form once again will be a choice that you will not regret.

When it comes to your Mental diet it focuses on bio roles. "Bio" means "life" in Greek. So basically your bio role means your life role. Looking into your bio-role dynamics, this deals with how the roles you play affect your daily life. It also looks into how you can step into a new lifestyle that includes you being thinner, healthier and happier than you are in your overweight, out of shape and unhealthy lifestyle. You know that at this point in your life you are not happy with the way you are living—if you were happy you probably would not be reading this book for starters. I know, speaking from my own personal experience, I always felt that I was a skinny person trapped inside an overweight body. When I began to change my way of living, giving up many of my bad eating habits, and adding exercise into my life—it was not easy to make changes—even though I knew they were for the better. I can say when I began to lose the excess weight it was so exhilarating to see bit by bit my skinny me finally being released. I know that you too can make this change—trade the overweight version in for the healthy version—you will have the best natural high from the experience when you begin to reap the benefits from your challenge.

Start by making small changes and shake up your bio role. Just because you are making small changes does not mean they are not important. The more positive changes you make in your life, even small ones, the will contribute to you weakening your old role's that grip you. It is important that you are willing to let go of your belief that you are doomed forever to be overweight and unhappy. At this point you need to begin to be willing to let go of your old lifestyle habits. If you don't let go of the belief that you are doomed—you are never going to be successful with any diet plan, you will just continue to sabotage any attempts at personal change. You need to be willing to consider that it is indeed possible that you can change.

Preparing for "D-Day"

There are a few things that you should do when you are preparing for D-Day. First you should be specific about what day will be your start date. Make sure to have a real clear picture of what your present role is. Write down about some of your beliefs about your eating habits and choice of foods. Take a moment to try and imagine how you would like to see yourself or imagine how you will look at the end of your challenge. Look for a role model, someone that can inspire you through those tough times ahead. Think of a new trait that you would really love to adopt. Think of an old trait that you want to toss in the rubbish bin.

For years Behaviourists have been saying that "you are how you act." But how you act can be changed. Try to think like a person that is thin and in shape, and act like you think they would act. Use your imagination to really get into the role. Then see the world through the eyes of a person that is not overweight, healthy both physically and mentally. Allow yourself to relate to and feel these things from the healthy person's perspective. You can build your new life role bit by bit and take down and get rid of your old role—trading it in for the healthy skinnier version! You are now ready to begin making your journey plans to building your new healthier role in life! Good luck and happy travels during your journey!

Conclusion

I hope that you will find the collection of healthy recipes, meal planner, exercises and along with other advice and suggestions useful to you on your journey towards that healthier lifestyle that you are seeking. You are heading in the right direction—making a great first step towards your new role as a person living a happier healthier lifestyle—by simply downloading this book. It shows that you are serious in wanting to make changes in your lifestyle. Keep in mind that Rome was not built in a day and either will your new lifestyle. It is going to take great personal commitment from you and the desire to truly want to reach your goals. Once you have made the mental decision to be willing to believe that you can change your lifestyle—then things are really going to start going your way in life.

The beginning of your journey is believing in yourself, that you can complete and succeed at your personal challenge. I wish you great success and happiness—you deserve to be healthy and happy in life! Be good to yourself—by starting to take care of yourself better by providing yourself with a healthy diet, exercise and mental peace of mind. I hope that you will find my books content a good guide and a sense of comfort in helping you to map out your journey towards your healthier life!

Made in the USA
Las Vegas, NV
14 October 2022

57273111R00036